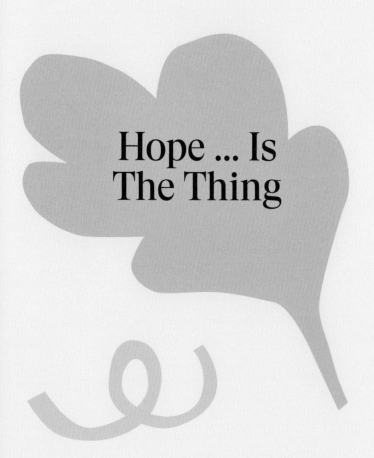

Hope ... Is
The Thing

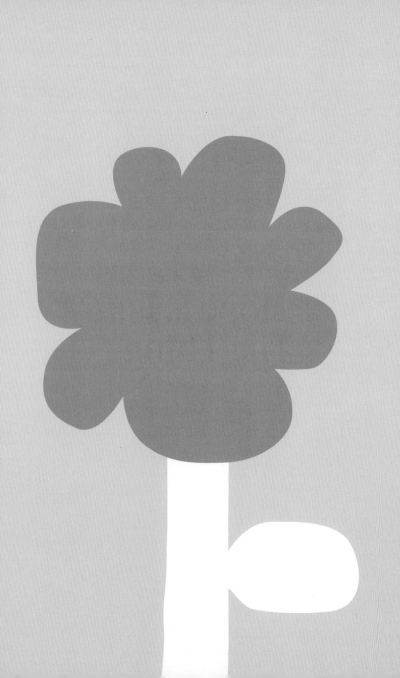

Susan Elizabeth Clark

Hope... is the thing

How to keep going, no matter what you are facing

OH EDITIONS

Hope fought hard to stay alive. Even when you thought it was beaten to nothing, burned to ashes, drowned deep, still it flickered away, waiting to be found again.

Juliet Marillier

DEN OF WOLVES

Hope is the thing with feathers —

That perches in the soul —

And sings the tune
without the words —

And never stops — at all —

Excerpt from '"Hope" is the thing with feathers'
by Emily Dickinson (1830—1886)

Introduction

What does the idea of Hope mean to you? Is it a fragile and frustratingly ephemeral idea that surfaces only to disappear again, almost as soon as you've felt its uplifting promise? Or do you think Hope could be something more substantial, robust even, and a welcome fixture in your life?

What if Hope was something you could, literally, 'will' into taking centre stage in all your actions and decisions. Would that make you happier and more optimistic about what lies ahead?

In her poem, '"Hope" is the thing with feathers,' Emily Dickinson likens Hope to a small bird that will sing and sing and sing: come rain, or shine, or snow, or storms. It is steadfast, courageous and noble; it is a metaphor we can all understand for Hope with a capital 'H'.

In that same spirit of courage and fortitude, *Hope ... Is The Thing* is the little book that reminds us that — whatever circumstances we may be facing — Hope enables us to carry on.

Let's celebrate the Hope we already have in our lives and learn how we can easily invite more in.

Without Hope, our lives
would be poorer and the world
would be darker; we'd find it harder
to remember that the rainbow
follows the storm.

Without Hope, we'd sometimes
feel we were trudging reluctantly
through the endless days ahead.

We All Need Hope

Hope is 'the thing' none of us would want to live without. It gets us up in the morning and carries us through good and bad times

With Hope, we can confidently put one foot in front of the other each and every day; moving forward with excited anticipation and positivity as our individual life path unfolds.

Hope is the Great Motivator!

With Hope, we can work together to create that better world we imagine for ourselves, our children and others.

To have Hope is to want an outcome that makes your life better: it makes a tough situation more bearable and also improves our lives.

Envisioning a better future will motivate you to take the steps you need to take to make it happen.

Hope lies in dreams, in imagination, and in the courage of those who dare to make dreams into reality.

Jonas Salk
SCIENTIST

Never underestimate
the power of hope.

Hope fuels us with the energy
and power to go forward.

Adèle Basheer
PHILOSOPHER & BUSINESSWOMAN

In the Hope Store Cupboard

What you'll need to get started on
actively inviting Hope — with a capital 'H' —
into your life:

An open mind.

An open heart.

A yoga or other non-slip
fitness map to practice some
simple and safe postures
that help open the Third Eye
(your body's psychic energy
centre) so you can manifest
the outcome of your greatest
Hopes and dreams.

A small candle or tea light for
the yogic practice of candle
gazing: to focus your mind
on Hope and to manifest it
in 'Magickal' ways.

A favourite journal,
dedicated solely to
a celebration of Hope.

Dried bay leaves.

Colouring pencils and
drawing paper.

We must vote for hope, vote for life, vote for a brighter future for all of our loved ones.

Ed Markey

LAWYER & POLITICIAN

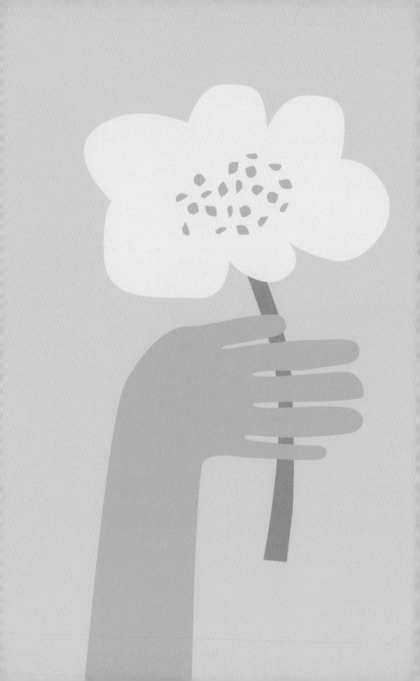

CHAPTER ONE

The Gift of Hope

Hope. It's a little word but one that carries so much weight.

Hope costs nothing and means everything.

Like those wise humans who shine a light on what it means to be truly Hopeful, champion it in the lives of others. If, say, someone you know and care about gets good news or recovers from an illness, acknowledge how Hopeful they must now feel moving forwards.

Turn into a Hope super-sleuth and don't just wait for it to show itself — search it out, in your own life and the lives of others. It will be a pleasure to do.

I throw wishes out into the night
and wait for stars to catch them.

Christy Ann Martine
WRITER & POET

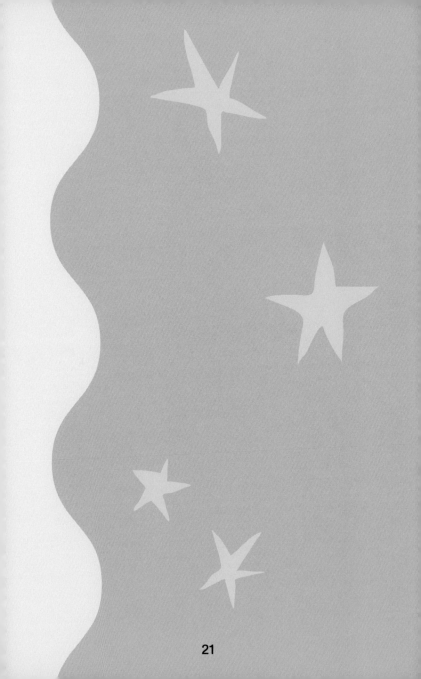

The Story of Hope

In Greek mythology, the beautiful Pandora carried a box of curses that may have been best left unopened; because when she opened the lid, out flew all of life's miseries: sickness, death, turmoil strife, jealousy, hatred, famine and passion.

These curses were said to be a punishment from the King of the ancient Greek gods — Zeus.

Zeus was furious that the other gods had given humans the power of fire.

But in a rare moment of softness, he added Hope to the mix.

And so, when all those curses had flown, Hope was left in Pandora's box to help humanity to face life's miseries.

It is because of hope that you suffer. It is through hope that you change things.

Maxime Lagacé

ICE HOCKEY PLAYER

Finding Hope

Scholars still debate whether Hope was meant as a blessing or a curse. There are those who argue that leaving humans with Hope was cruel: because even when the odds are against us, and reality tells us there's no point carrying on, we do anyway — in Hope of a better outcome.

Others believe facing life's challenges and miseries with no Hope at all would feel very bleak.

I choose to believe Hope is one of our truly great blessings.

In the exercise overleaf, you'll make your own 'Pandora's Box' with Hope safely tucked inside.

This will help you to see how Hope is already supporting you.

EXERCISE

In your Hope Journal, list three
hurtful things that have happened in your
life. (These will probably be things you'd like
to keep a lid on.)

You may have had your heart broken
or been passed over for a job; been trolled
or bullied or misjudged online.

Now ask yourself
'How did Hope help me?'

How does Hope help
heal a broken heart?

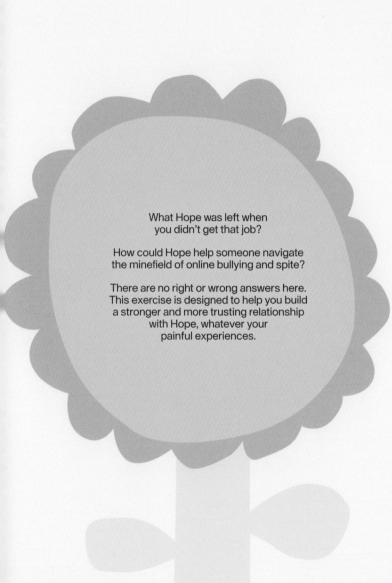

What Hope was left when
you didn't get that job?

How could Hope help someone navigate
the minefield of online bullying and spite?

There are no right or wrong answers here.
This exercise is designed to help you build
a stronger and more trusting relationship
with Hope, whatever your
painful experiences.

A positive statement propels hope towards a better future, it builds up your faith, and that of others, and promotes change.

Jan Dargatz
SELF-HELP WRITER

Hope is a waking dream.

Aristotle
PHILOSOPHER

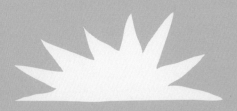

What Do You Hope For?

Part I: In your Hope Journal, list three things you are hoping for right now.

Don't second-guess yourself or talk yourself down. Be honest and daring — if you are hoping for something to happen, write it down

Choose just one of those three Hopes and, in your journal, write a short story about life after it comes true.

Dream big, your story can be as crazy as you like! Imagine all the wildest possibilities that can happen if that particular Hope comes to pass.

Part II: You've imagined a wonderful future — now we need to think about how you can make that Hope a reality.

In your Hope Journal, write down some steps you can take to turn this Hope into a dream-come-true.

Answer the following:

What I can do today?

What I can do this week?

What I can do this month?

What I can do this year?

If your Hope is about work, you can start looking for new opportunities. One of the first big steps will be to update your CV and register with online recruiters.

Another step is to put the word out amongst your family and friend networks. Tell them what you are hoping for: to find a new direction, to work more or less, or to make more time to do what you love.

Remember, there is no right or wrong. Only what feels right for you.

If your Hope is about Love and finding someone authentic to share your life with, try stepping away from dating apps with all their limitations. Instead, join a group — either online or in real life — to share an activity you love or learn something completely new.

This could be writing.

Or community singing.

Or a fun general knowledge quiz night.

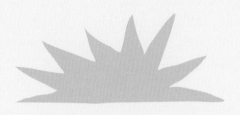

Optimism is the faith that leads to achievement. Nothing can be done without hope and confidence.

Helen Keller
DISABILITY RIGHTS & POLITICAL ACTIVIST

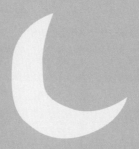

Let your hopes, not your hurts,
shape your future.

Robert H. Schuller
MOTIVATIONAL SPEAKER

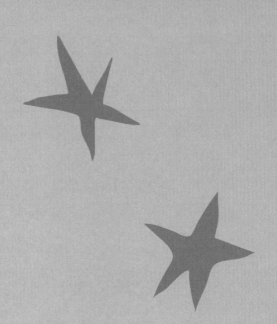

CHAPTER TWO

The Power of Hope

Hope is the belief things will work, especially when it seems otherwise. It helps you stay calm and peaceful when something less than desirable emerges.

Hope believes you will get through it.

Hope remembers the times you made it through.

Hope teams with Faith and believes in the impossible.

Anon

We All Share Hope

You may be strangers, passing by each other at a railway station or sitting at opposite ends of a café, but when you both got up this morning you did so sharing a belief in Hope.

You can't touch it, smell it, buy it or prove it exists.

But we all know it does.

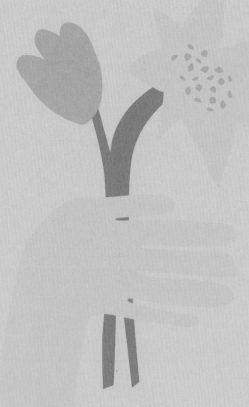

One of the greatest powers of Hope is that, like love, we share a collective understanding of its importance.

When we share a belief in an idea, we can start to create unbreakable bonds built on that understanding.

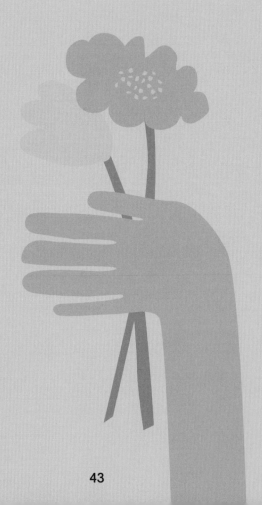

A person can do incredible
things if he or she has enough hope.

Shannon J. Butcher
AUTHOR

They say a person needs just three things to be truly happy in this world: someone to love, something to do, and something to hope for.

Tom Bodett
AUTHOR & RADIO HOST

Symbols of Hope

Flower Symbols

Floriology — the use of flowers to convey a message or a meaning

In the Victorian Era, flowers held symbolic meanings. People sent coded messages to each other — including ones of love and admiration and even admonishment — by sending a posy.

We may have lost this wonderful language of flowers from our culture today, but you don't have to dig too deep to find out what flower your Victorian ancestor would have known was a symbol of Hope...

...that flower is the humble winter Snowdrop

Plant a small pot of snowdrops to keep
on the windowsill — this will serve as
a reminder that spring always
follows winter.

Plant a second pot and give it to someone
who is having a hard time right now and is
struggling — it may allow them to hang on to
the Hope that things will get better for them.

Animal Symbols

Esoteric traditions and indigenous cultures often attach symbolic meaning to the spirits of animals.
    The animal that is symbolic of Hope is the common Blackbird.

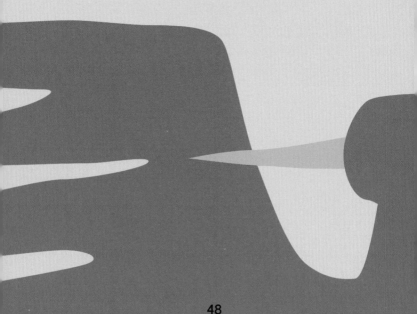

Blackbird: The only bird to sing before dawn breaks.

How Hopeful and trusting is that?

If you live in a country (or the countryside) where one of the signs of spring is the sight of a field of newborn lambs, you will likely have felt the jolt of Hope this bucolic scene can trigger.

New life — in animal or plant form — is a reminder that life is a cycle and that just as night follows day, good times will follow bad.

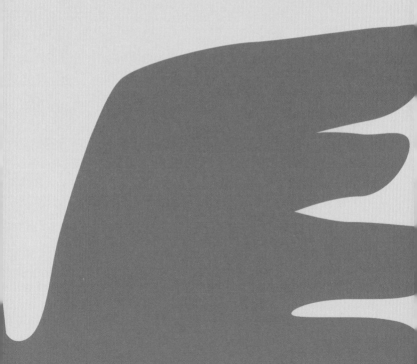

Colour Symbols

Yellow is for Hope, happiness and spontaneity.

To help you feel more Hopeful: buy a yellow mug, fill a vase with yellow flowers, or keep a citrine crystal in your pocket

Once cleansed*, your crystal will attract more Hope and Hopeful opportunities into your life. It will remind you, when you wake each morning, to stay Hopeful and optimistic in all that you think and do.

*Crystals absorb energy which is what makes them so useful in energy work, but this also means it is important to cleanse any crystal that is new to you and your home. We do this to make sure we are not susceptible to any energy it has absorbed from others. You can cleanse your citrine crystal by washing it with distilled water.

Once you choose Hope,
anything's possible.

Christopher Reeve
ACTOR

Rainbows

The rainbow has been adopted all over the world as a powerful symbol of Hope.

It came to the fore once more during the Coronavirus Pandemic when, in some countries,
it was used to celebrate key workers.

An 'adapted' rainbow has been a potent symbol of Hope for the LBGT+ community for several decades.

The six-stripe Pride rainbow flag dates back to 1978 when it was created by San Francisco-based Queer artist, Gilbert Baker.

The flag was originally eight stripes but has evolved over time, and today its colours are:

Red – for Life

Orange – for Healing

Yellow – for Sunlight

Green – for Nature

Blue – for Harmony

Purple – for Spirit

Rainbow Babies

Families who have suffered the terrible grief that follows the death of a baby often refer to subsequent children as their 'Rainbow Babies'.

They simply mean that the safe birth and survival of these children represent the sunnier days that follow a terrible storm of grief.

Rainbow Babies are the embodiment of Hope at its most courageous.

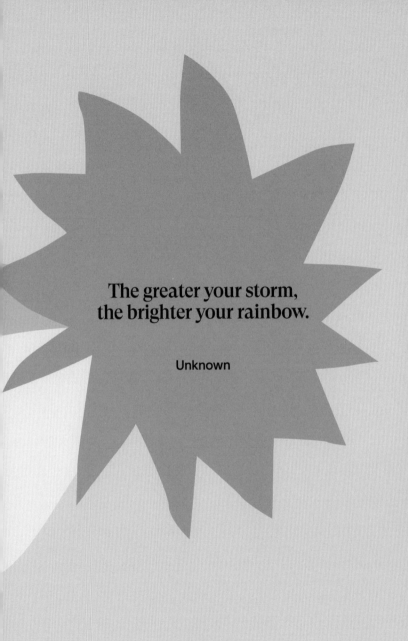

The greater your storm,
the brighter your rainbow.

Unknown

Hope Is Believing

Hope is not about wishing
something were true.
Hope is an actual belief.

AFFIRMATION

I believe in Hope.

I trust Hope.

I know Hope will pull me through,
whatever dark times I may face.

Healing Hearts and Minds

Psychologists, and others working in the field of mental health and wellness, know the true power of Hope.

They will tell you that Hope, more than any other characteristic or quality, differentiates the victim from the survivor.

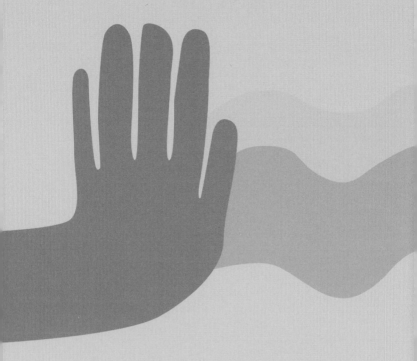

This is not a judgement but a clinically observed fact.
If someone has lost all Hope, and never finds it again,
the road back to health and happiness may be lost to
them forever.
Hope plays a powerful role in healing hearts and minds.

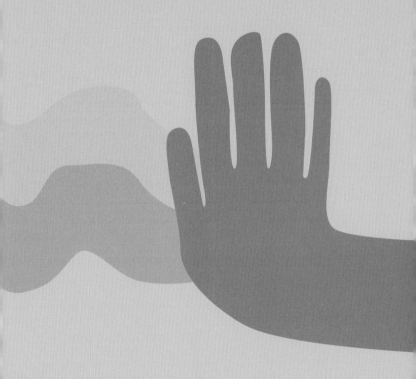

Far away there in the sunshine are my highest aspirations. I may not reach them but I can look up and see their beauty, believe in them, and try to follow them.

Louisa May Alcott
AUTHOR

People usually consider hope among the most wondrous of gifts: it keeps us going when we want to quit and makes possible victories that seem unattainable.

Dr Alex Lickerman
AUTHOR OF *THE UNDEFEATED MIND*

AFFIRMATION

Hope comes from the heart, not the brain.

That makes Hope a truly loving
quality — and it's the reason why you
cannot separate Love from Hope.

Hope tells you that you can endure.

That means Hope will give you the strength
to face whatever comes your way, even when
you believe you will not survive it.

Hope Rises

In her final speech as First Lady, Michelle Obama talked about the power of Hope.

Here's what she said:

'It is our fundamental belief in the power of hope that has allowed us to rise above the voices of doubt and division, of anger and fear that we have faced in our own lives and the life of this country.'

And Michelle was not the only First Lady to talk about Hope. Her predecessor, Eleanor Roosevelt, who was First Lady between 1933 and 1945, said this:

'Surely, in the light of history, it is more intelligent to hope rather than to fear, to try rather than not to try. For one thing, we know beyond all doubt: Nothing has ever been achieved by the person who says, "It can't be done."'

Awakening Hope

Everyone Hopes for something and with this simple exercise you'll learn what you are hoping for today, tomorrow, next week and next year.

You can extrapolate as far into the future as you want.

When you have finished the exercise, take some time to imagine the things you are hoping for coming to pass.

In your Hope Journal, finish the
following statements:

Today I am Hoping ...

Tomorrow I am Hoping ...

Next week, I Hope ...

Next year I Hope ...

Few things in the world are more powerful than a positive push. A smile. A world of optimism and Hope. A 'You Can Do It' when things get tough.

Richard M. DeVos
BUSINESSMAN

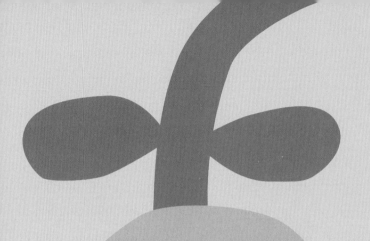

AFFIRMATION

I believe in Hope

I believe in Hope

I believe in Hope

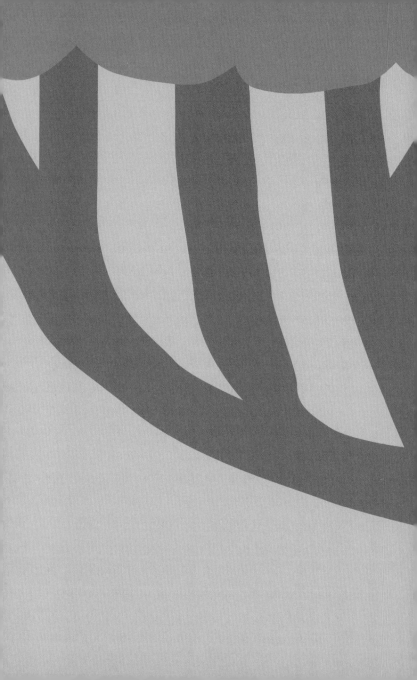

CHAPTER THREE

Circles of Hope

The birth of every baby — including you — is the Universe's ultimate celebration of Hope. In this chapter, we will explore how the thing we are all really made of — aside from flesh and bones — is Hope with a capital 'H'.

Bringing the gifts that my ancestors gave, I am the dream and the hope of the slave. I rise. I rise. I rise.

Albert Schweitzer

HUMANITARIAN

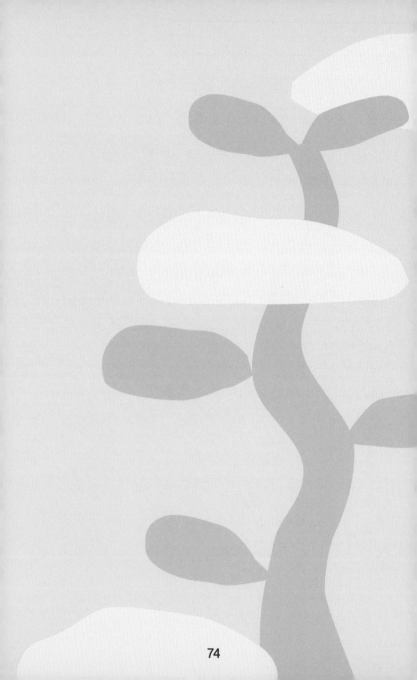

You are the fairy tale
told by your ancestors.

Jean-Jacques Rousseau
PHILOSOPHER

You are a Triumph of Hope

You are going to need your powers of imagination for this exercise *; it is all about honouring the strong threads of Hope that weave your life back to the lives of your ancestors. Imagine how many people and how much Hope this represents.

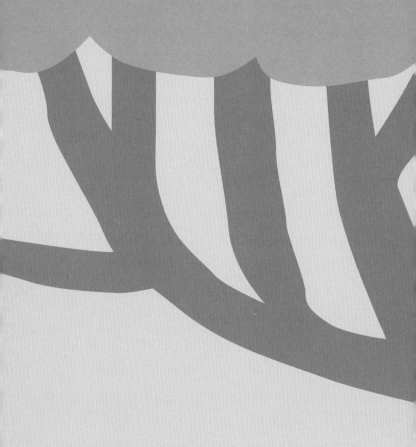

We all have two parents, two sets of Grandparents, four sets of Great Grandparents and eight sets of Great-Great Grandparents. So, that's 16 people just four generations back!

*This is a powerful exercise, before you begin it, take a minute to think about its potential impact on you.

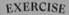

Ancestral Hopes

Let's start with a yoga exercise that helps to open your Third Eye — an energy centre located in the middle of your forehead, just above your eyebrows — so you can 'see' all those threads of Hope that connect you back to the people you come from.

**You will need: a quiet place, a candle,
a favourite blanket or shawl**

Sit in a position you find most comfortable, in a quiet place
where you can focus without distraction

Light a candle or tea light and place it in your line of vision.
Sit quietly, listening to the rise and fall of your breath, as
you stare at the flickering flame. Keep your gaze on the
flame and try not to blink.

At some point, your vision will begin to blur a little. You may
also feel a tingling in the middle of your forehead but don't
worry if you don't feel anything.

This is when your Third Eye will open and instead of using
your normal vision, you can now tune in to your psychic
powers. We all have these powers, sometimes it just takes
a little practice to kickstart our connection to them.

As your Third Eye opens, picture one of your ancestors —
someone without whom you would not have the gift of life.

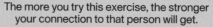

The more you try this exercise, the stronger your connection to that person will get.

If you know your ancestor's name then use it here; if not, just imagine this person's energy and the joy and Hope they felt when a new baby was born into their family — your family!

It doesn't matter if you don't know names. Your Third Eye will help connect you to your ancestral energy and the joy surrounding the birth that links, like a fence, directly to your own birth.

Spend some time imagining, experiencing and fully feeling the joy of all this shared Hope. If you have a child or children yourself, or there are other children in your family, then take yourself back to the happiness you felt when they were safely born — and revel in the Hope of that moment.

Congratulations, you've just made your first connection to your own family's Circle of Hope.

When you are ready, snuff out the candle and record this experience in your Hope Journal.

Hope is an embrace of the unknown.

Rebecca Solnit
SOCIAL CHANGE ACTIVIST

I Rise

Imagine the challenges all of your ancestors — including your parents — had to rise against and overcome in order for you to inherit Hope and the gift of life.

    In your Hope journal write down three of their successes if you know them; if not, imagine three ways one of your ancestors would have faced and overcome hardship based on the historical times in which they were born.

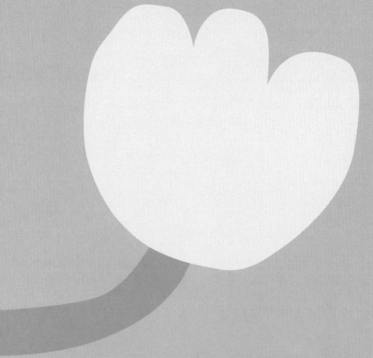

I Rise Too ...

In your Hope Journal, list three ways in which you have risen to overcome challenges in your own life.

Now write one short paragraph about how you found Hope in each of those darker times you've listed.

The Path Unwinding

Find a big bold crayon or pen and in your Hope Journal write down four really big Hopes that you have for yourself for the next two years.

These need to be BIG HOPES so use BIG WRITING.

Use the list opposite and write as much as you like when you are describing each of these four BIG HOPES.

Really imagine yourself living in a life that has been changed by each of these Hopes.

How will you feel once each Hope has come to fruition?

Relish that feeling for each of the four Hopes.

1. I Hope to have ...

2. I Hope to see ...

3. I Hope to become ...

4. I Hope to help ...

Now carefully remove these pages from your Hope Journal and tuck them somewhere safe where you can forget about them.

Put an alert into your phone for the same day, in two years' time.

When you next see these pages, you'll have an even better understanding of how Hope is the trusty guide that accompanies us as our own unique life path unwinds.

When you were baptised*,
your ancestors looked down
on you with Hope.

Henry B Eyring

*You may not have been baptised but welcomed into the world by your family in some
other traditional or meaningful way. However it was that you've been welcomed, the
invisible thread back to your ancestors and their Hopes and dreams remains unbroken.

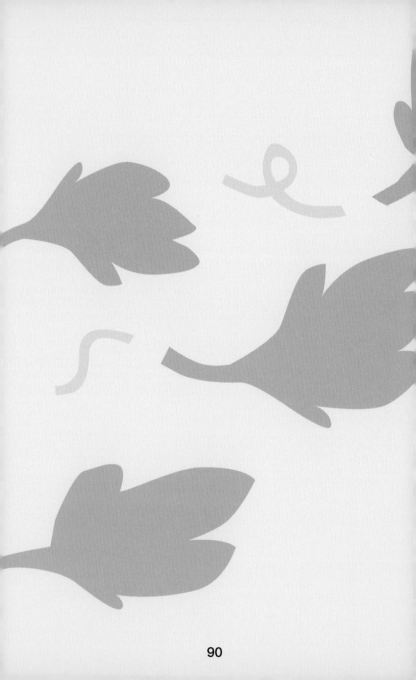

Our ancestors knew that healing comes in circles and cycles. One generation carries the pain so that the next can live and heal. One cannot live without the other, each is the other's hope, meaning and strength.

Gemma B. Benton

Hopes and Dreams

If you really want to intimately know someone — a love, a newly-discovered ancestor, an old flame — ask yourself not 'who are they?' or 'what do they do?'; but the much more revealing question: 'what are or were their Hopes and dreams?'.

We can't separate our Hopes from our dreams so once you understand one, you know the other.

Try and develop your ability to 'hear'
what someone Hopes for, even if they never tell
you with words. Think of someone you care about
and ask yourself:

What do you think is their biggest
Hope for themselves, right now?

What do you think is their biggest
Hope for the planet?

Put your answers to the test by asking them these
questions the next time you meet or speak.

It is an honour if they share their greatest Hopes
and dreams with you. How close are your insights
to what they reveal?

We all have an unexpected reserve of strength inside us that emerges when life puts us to the test.

Isabel Allende
WRITER

It is in the roots, not the branches,
that a tree's greatest strength lies.

Matshona Dhliwayo

PHILOSOPHER

Hope is Free

The first step in making Hope the foundation of your life is to remember it is an equal opportunity resource that isn't dependent on your income, your IQ or your looks.

It is free, it's available to you all of the time and it's yours for the taking!

When you need more of it, don't hang about shyly at the back of the queue — there is no queue. Go and get as much as you need to get you through ...

There is nothing passive about being Hopeful and sharing Hope with other people.

Being Hopeful is an active choice and one you can choose whenever you need it.

Choosing Hope every time things don't go your way, or you run into something outside your control that makes you unhappy is just that — your choice.

How Hope Works

It can be tempting to confuse Hope with 'wishful thinking' but psychologists who study Hope say the two are not at all the same.

'Wishing is ubiquitous but it can be kind of an escape from reality,' says Jon G. Allen, a professor of psychology and behavioural sciences. 'Hope is different because it has to do with facing reality.

As I see it, it's about staying in the game.'

Hope is a Choice

Here's a choice: do you look at life as a glass half-full or a glass half-empty person?

People who look at reality from the perspective of the glass being half-full are more Hopeful than those who think the glass is half-empty and likely to stay that way!

Hope Likes Company

Hope likes company and the more you share Hope with others, the more it bounces right back to you.

Hope thrives on good and supportive social connections.

Healthcare workers know only too well the value of Hope; they report that patients who lose Hope feel invisible and alone.

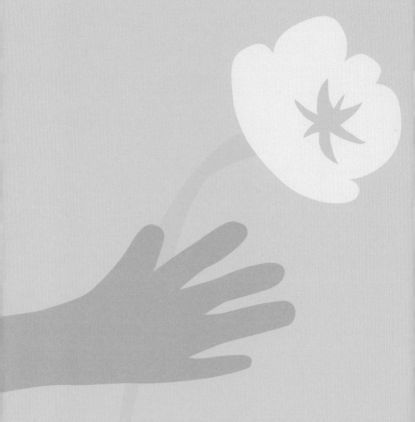

If you can change someone's feeling of being forgotten and isolated, by making sure they feel seen and noticed and not on their own; then you can help them feel better about what lies ahead.

Once you give them Hope, there's no place for hopelessness.

Mind the GAP

In order to bring more Hope into your life, you need to know about the 'GAP' which stands for:

Goals

Agency

Pathways

The late American psychologist, Charles R. Snyder, who was a pioneer of Hope research at the University of Kansas developed the GAP model of Hope.

You already know what is meant by goals, but agency may be a newer idea to you. Put simply, it means you have the power to shape your life and make things happen to achieve your goals.

Pathways is just another word for how you get there (you can think of this as being the same as steps or choices) and what routes you take.

Hope can be a powerful force.
Maybe there's no actual magic in it, but
when you know what you hope for most
and hold it like a light within you, you can
make things happen, almost like magic.

Laini Taylor
FANTASY WRITER

Hope is the companion of power, and mother of success; for who so hopes strongly has within him the gift of miracles.

Samuel Smiles
POLITICAL REFORMER

Hope and Success

Being Hopeful is a better predictor of success in life than academic achievement, intelligence or personality.

Researchers at Leicester University in the UK tracked college students for three years and reported that those who expressed the most Hope went on to the greatest academic success.

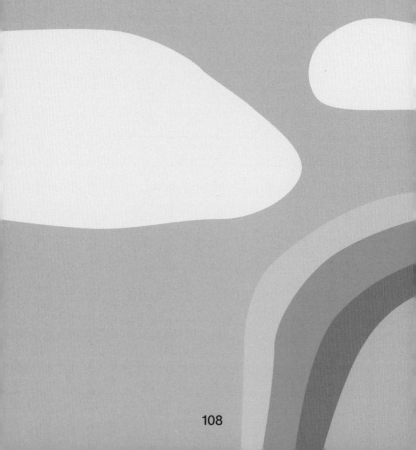

On the other side of the pond, researchers looking at the role of Hope in workplace productivity reported that Hopeful workers did, on average, the equivalent of one more day's work in a week than a less Hopeful work colleague.

CHAPTER FOUR

Keeping Faith With Hope

Think of someone you know — a friend, a family member, a work colleague — who stayed Hopeful against overwhelming odds.

What do they have that keeps even the smallest flicker of Hope alive when all seems lost?

You can't see the thing they rely on to stay Hopeful, because you can't see, touch or feel Faith — with a capital 'F'.

People who have Faith know that Hope will get them through. They show the rest of us that strength comes from the courage of our convictions.

So, what if you can't see it or sell it, buy it or bottle it? That doesn't mean it — Faith — doesn't exist.

Word which the finger of
God has written on the brow
of every man — Hope!

Victor Hugo

NOVELIST

Hope is a Blessing

Remember when we talked about how Hope stayed in Pandora's box — we said that scholars still debate whether Hope was supposed to be a blessing or a curse?

There will be times in all of our lives when Hope can seem false or like an absent friend.

Maybe your partner falls sick and doesn't recover. Or perhaps you don't get that dream job.

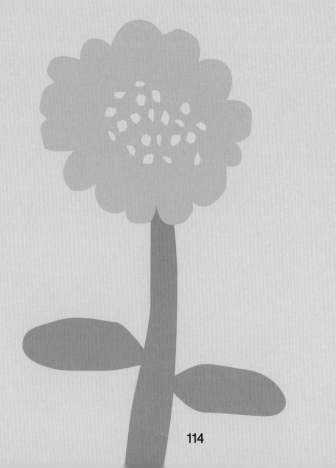

Yes, Hope can help us deal with the most crushing of disappointments, but Hope can also feel fragile.

So, what can you do when it feels like Hope has forgotten you?

How do you get her back?

Keep the Faith. When it feels like all Hope is gone for good you can and will get her back.

And even if you have to 'fake it until you make it', one day you will look back at the hard times and understand Hope never once left your side — not even when everything felt and looked hopeless.

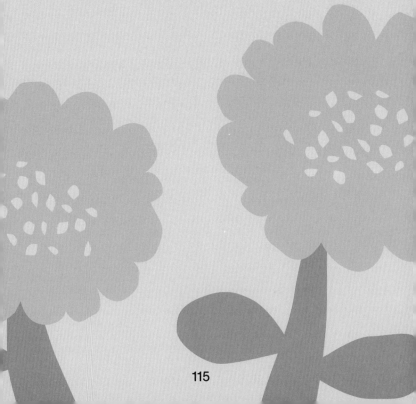

Man can live 40 days without food, three days without water, eight minutes without air, but only one second without hope.

Cam Taylor-Britt
ATHLETE

We cry from pain, from loss and from loneliness, but mostly we cry because we still have hope, and because we can still find joy, even on the darkest and coldest of winter nights.

Courtney M. Privett
AUTHOR

Hope and Despair

These two feelings are the opposite sides of the same coin.

Think about it.

If we didn't feel Hope, we
wouldn't feel despair.

Without despair, we wouldn't need Hope.

This is why the question of whether Hope is a blessing or a curse for humankind is such a testing one.

I think the bigger question though is: how on earth can we manage feelings of despair if we don't have Hope to pull us through and out the other side of darker times in our lives?

How does anyone who has had their heart broken find the courage to try again?

They find it — the courage — lurking just out of sight, behind Hope

Along this path of darkness there's always light waiting to be seen by our daunted hearts.

Our heart is gifted to see this light.

It may be hiding behind those circumstances that we encounter; in a stranger we just met at an unexpected place; a family who has been always there, but you just ignored because of your imperfect relationship with them; it might be a long-time friend you have or a friend you just met.

Open your heart and you will see how blessed you are to have them all in your life. Sometimes they are the light that shines your path in some dark phases of life.

Don't lose hope!

Chanda Kaushik
WRITER

Pinning Your Hopes

Hope can feel fragile and ephemeral —
a fleeting feeling that rushes by so fast it can
be hard to grab hold of for long enough to power
us through the darker times.

Maybe that's why we talk of 'pinning our Hopes'
on something. We have a strong need to anchor
ourselves to a positive feeling that can help us
navigate difficult times.

In this little exercise, we're not 'pinning the tail on
the donkey'; instead, we're pinning our Hope(s)
onto something solid that we can hold on to.

Symbols are a powerful reminder of our deepest Hopes
and dreams.

If what you Hope for most this year is true love, then draw
a heart and stick it in your journal or pin it somewhere you will
see it every day — like a fridge door.

If you Hope for (and dream of) more meaningful work,
imagine what kind of work this will be and draw or fashion
a symbol to represent taking a step towards work that matters
to your heart.

Let your imagination and your creativity soar —
see if you can identify and create a symbol for at least
six different Hopes.

A Tree of Hope(s)

Once you have your symbols you need something to 'pin' them on!

We're using the phrase 'pin' metaphorically here, so you can tie or tape or stick your symbols however you wish and on to whatever you wish.

One nice idea is to make your own symbolic Tree of Hope using an old branch or stick.

Or you can simply tack your symbols to the mirror in your bedroom or tie them all to a long piece of twine or string to make a laundry-style banner of Hope.

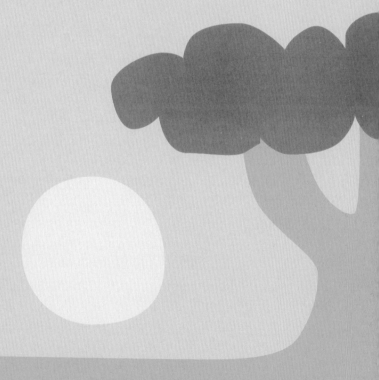

Whichever creative solution you choose, make sure you display your 'pinned' Hopes somewhere you can easily see them every day.

In fact, make this a proud display, not something you hide away.

It will act as a great conversation point with others and encourage them to talk about their Hope(s) and Dreams too. Which, as we discovered earlier, is a great way of getting to know people better and on a more meaningful level.

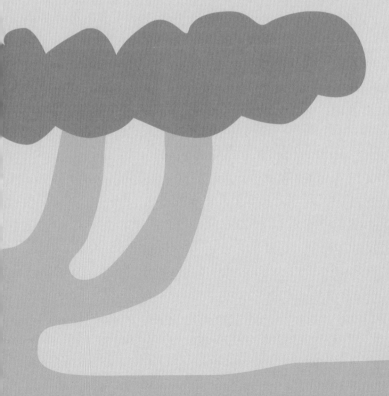

Hope is a match in a dark tunnel, a moment of light, just enough to reveal the path ahead and ultimately the way out.

Dr Judith Rich

You can always see a light around the hopeful people and darkness around the hopeless! And what better shield can you have than having a light around you in the dusky times?

Mehmet Murat Ildan

WRITER

Building Hope

It may sometimes feel as if Hope was 'given out' as a genetic gift to some and not to others but that's really not true.

Yes, some people seem more optimistic and able to bounce back from disappointment, full of Hope and even hoping against Hope. They aren't privy to some hidden secret that was handed out when you were looking the other way, or standing in the glass-half-empty queue.

They've just mastered the 1, 2, 3 Steps to building up Hope as a life tool and I'm going to share them with you here.

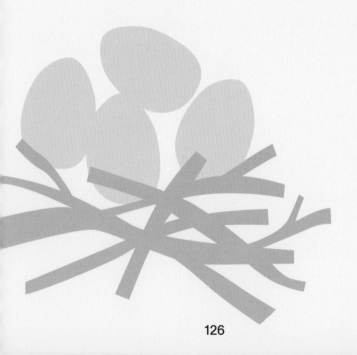

Psychologists have discovered that when faced with a crisis, less Hopeful people shut down whereas more Hopeful people take whatever action is needed to help them cope.

And we're not talking a bunch of idealistic 'Pollyannas' here. Because above all else, Hopeful people are pragmatic.

They know they need to work on making Hope(s) a reality and they will be the first to roll up their sleeves ...

Getting Hope

Here are the 1, 2, 3 Steps to building Hope, getting Hope, keeping Hope and staying more Hopeful — whatever crisis you may be facing.

Step 1
If you want more Hope,
act like you already have it.
Just fake it until you make it!

Step 2
Come up with multiple ways
to get past the obstacles blocking
your goals so if one way doesn't
work, try another.

Step 3
Get real and set multiple
goals. Then, if one dream
doesn't manifest you've
always got another.

Learn the Art of Re-Goaling

I'm going to talk about something very sad to show you what I mean by this.

Think about how the parents of a terminally ill child must, over time, shift their Hopes and goals.

Terminal means no cure and so there will be only one tragic end to this story.

What the parents must do is shift their 'Hope' to a new goal — one where the priority is to help their child live out their remaining time as comfortably and as peacefully as possible.

Sometimes, holding on to Hope will mean letting go of our biggest dreams in order to create new ones.

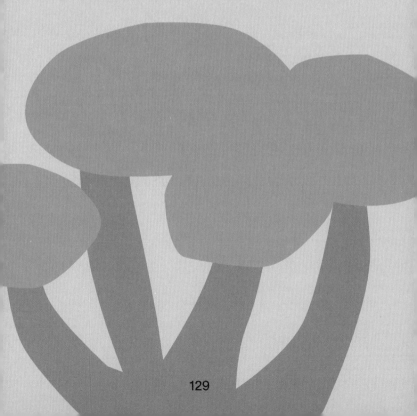

Hope is a renewable option:
If you run out of it at the end
of the day, you get to start over
in the morning.

Barbara Kingsolver
NOVELIST

Hope begins in the dark.
The stubborn hope that if you just show up
and try to do the right thing, the dawn will
come. You wait and watch and work: you
don't give up.

Anne Lamott
WRITER

Types of Hope

Understanding that there are different types of Hope can help you build more Hope into your day, your future and your outlook on life.

One easy way to categorise Hope, is to label it as being either a little 'Everyday Hope': like hoping it won't rain when you go out for a walk; or a 'Big Hope': like hoping nobody in your family will fall sick and die.

Psychologists have now defined seven different types of Hope.

Take a look at the different definitions and see if you can slot any of your current Hopes into these categories.

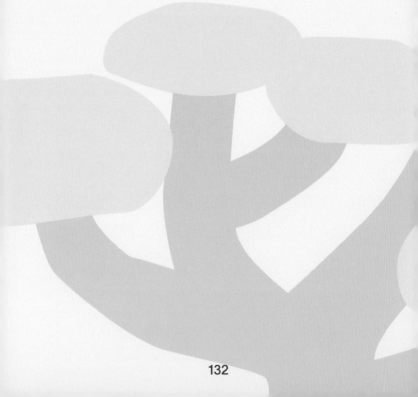

Inborn Hope

We all start out as children with Inborn Hope. We only lose it when bad things happen, and we begin to understand life may not always turn out how we Hoped it would.

The trick, or life hack, is to find your way to Mature Hope from Inborn Hope — which is what this little book will help you to do.

Mature Hope is the kind of Hope that waits for the outcome it desires.

Mature Hope also understands that sometimes, when things don't work out as we hoped, it leaves a space for another kind of magic to happen.

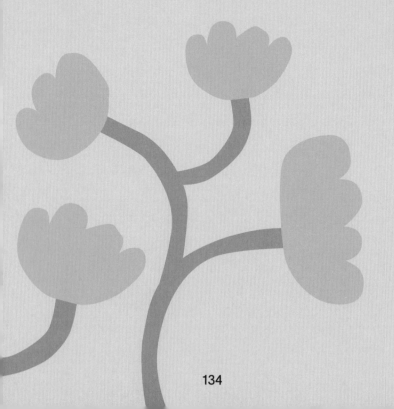

Chosen and Borrowed Hope

Chosen Hope is the Hope which persists in the face of adversity and overcomes the obstacles that undermine our Faith in Hope.

It may be choosing to Hope someone you love will survive a late-stage cancer diagnosis, even when you know the odds are stacked against them.

Chosen Hope can be a reflection of a person's natural disposition; it is true that some people seem to have a more 'glass half-full' approach to life than others. But even if you think 'glass-half-empty', you can still make a choice to find Hope when it is out of sight.

Borrowed Hope is the Hope we literally 'borrow' from someone else, but only if it comes from a place of love. Sometimes other people can see that good things lie in wait for us, even when we can't.

Bargainer's Hope

When the chips are down, we may find ourselves trading in Bargainer's Hope. We may hear a voice in our head saying, 'Just do this [one thing] and then what you want to happen will happen.'

There is nothing wrong with this type of Hope. I like to think of it as the teenage version of Hope, probably because teenagers are amongst the best 'bargainers' I have ever met!

However, this is not Hope in its mature form.

Bargaining is not a million miles from gambling and so there's always the risk the whole house of cards will come tumbling down — regardless of what you were hoping.

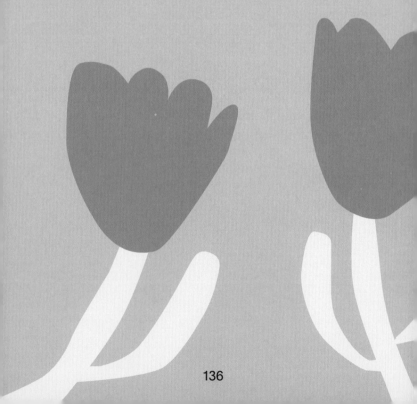

False and Unrealistic Hope

We've all had them at one time or another in our lives.
These are the kind of Hopes where we imagine we can
realise a desire or dream, without putting the work in.

Maybe we Hope we will be the best guitar player in
the world.

This would be a reasonable enough Hope, until we admit
we never practice. And that then makes it unrealistic.

False Hopes are just as silly. Maybe we Hope that if we
just think ourselves thinner, then one morning we will wake
up and it will be so.

We all know that to lose weight we have to move more
and eat less.

So, this easy-weight-loss false Hope is just a case
of wishful thinking.

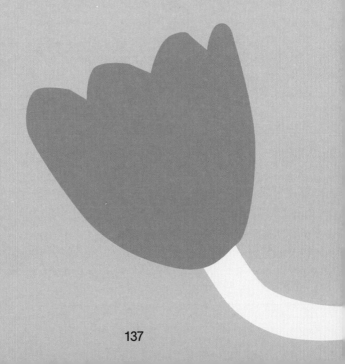

Mature Hope

We all start out as children with Inborn Hope. We only lose it when bad things happen, and we begin to understand life may not always turn out how we Hoped it would.

The trick/life hack is to find your way to Mature Hope from Inborn Hope — which is what this little book will help you do.

Mature Hope is the kind of Hope that can wait for the outcome it desires.

Mature Hope also understands that sometimes, when things don't work out as we hoped, it leaves a space for some other kind of magic to happen.

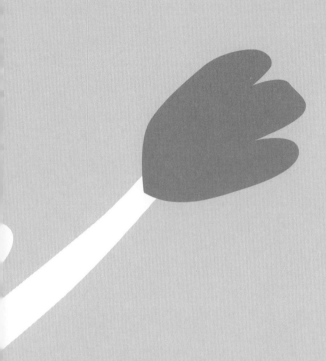

Hope and Faith

So now we know the way we keep Faith with Hope is by choosing to believe Hope will pull us through, whatever obstacles we may face.

Love is the source
And goal

Faith is the slow process
Of getting there

Hope is the willingness
To move forward
Without resolution

Richard Rohr
MEDITATION TEACHER

At the end of the day, all you need is Hope and Strength. Hope that it will get better and strength to hold on, until it does!

Unknown

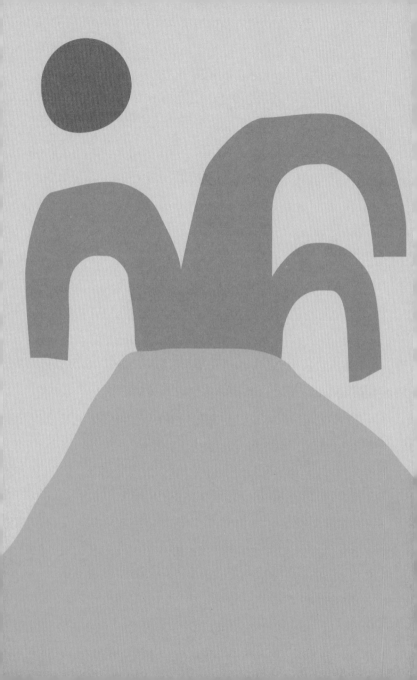

CHAPTER FIVE

Living In Hope

Hope has been keeping you company ever since it first showed up in your life. However quietly, Hope plays a key role in all the decisions you make — from who you love to where you work.

So, let's celebrate the almighty power of 'Living In Hope' and see for ourselves how Hope can move mountains — especially when we join with others to create a better world from shared dreams.

You can think of Hope as being just the same as the light from your torch when you are trying to find your way in the dark. Without it you may stumble; with it, you can see the way ahead and step purposefully towards the future.

The very least you can do in your life is figure out what you hope for. And the most you can do is live inside that hope. Not admire it from a distance but live right in it, under its roof.

Barbara Kingsolver

NOVELIST

Baby Steps ...

Without Hope, there is no 'What next?'

The true message of Hope is:

Keep going, no matter what.

Don't give up, no matter what.

Don't lose Hope, no matter what.

Instead, remember: This Too Shall Pass

When things get really bad, remember that it will not always be this way — this hard, this punishing, this soulless, this joyless. And remember too, there is a path through darkness when it comes; a path that is illuminated by your Hope.

This path is one you can trust. It has been well-trodden by the footsteps of others — so you are not alone.

This path is one of baby steps; one foot placed in front of the other.

It can sound glib to say just keep going but if you start by allowing yourself a glimmer of Hope for just a minute and then for, maybe, an hour, before long you'll be able to consider taking one morning or one afternoon at a time.

Remember, all you are doing is reminding yourself nothing stays the same forever, and so whatever the challenge you are facing, it too will pass.

Before long, you are managing one day at a time and by the time you can contemplate a week at a time, you are out of the crisis and walking purposefully again, with Hope at your side.

This Too Shall Pass

When we are in a place where it can be difficult to even believe in Hope, let alone connect to it, then these words may sound just like white noise.

So, with this exercise, we're going to experience the truth of this simple but powerful adage.

You cannot rush or boss it, but you can trust that if you do this exercise you will find respite. It helps you to work with, instead of fighting, against the painful feelings that are threatening to overwhelm you.

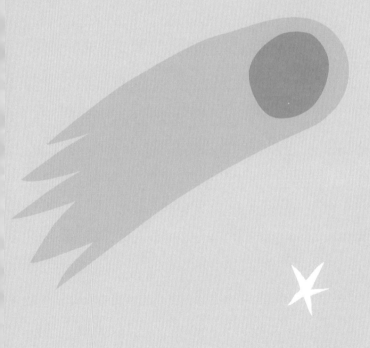

What Do You Hope For?

One Minute at a Time

Sit somewhere you wouldn't normally find yourself – on a wall outside, halfway up or down the stairs, on a rock on a beach. Take a breath and count up to a minute, slowly, in seconds. It doesn't matter if you come up short or overshoot, what matters is you survived!

One Hour at a Time

Set an alarm on your phone for precisely one hour from now.
As you set the alarm tell yourself: I am allowed to take a break from the
misery. Do something that used to make you happy and do it for the full hour.
Sing, draw, bake, walk, paint, read a book. The only rule is you must do this
alone, don't spend the hour texting friends or looking for other distractions
to get away from yourself. When the alarm goes off, stop whatever you were
doing. Draw a star in your journal by today's date. And accept, you survived.

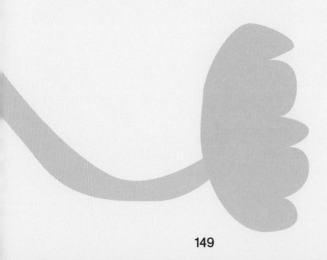

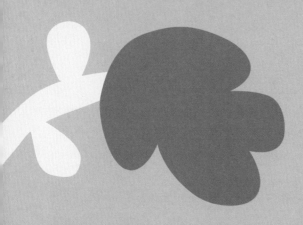

One Morning/Afternoon at a Time

Dress for the weather and go out. It does not matter where but take this trip alone. Walk, drive or cycle, it doesn't matter how you get to your destination. It doesn't even matter where your destination is. Just move. Move your body, feel your energy. Go out and stay out for a few hours, half a day.

Congratulations, you survived!

One Day at a Time

Before life crashed and Hope fled, what was your
favourite day of the week? Pick that day for this exercise.
Start the day with a treat: this could be a long bath, your favourite
breakfast or a trip to the local coffee shop.

It doesn't matter what you do, just treat yourself.

You may still be feeling disconnected from your 'before life'
and from the people who care about you, but this day is all about
you so put everything else to the side.

Do something that you used to enjoy as a child; if kicking
a ball was your thing, go to the park. If you liked scraping the cake bowl
once the mix was in the tin, make a cake but focus on the scraping.

This day is about you.

A day is a long time, and the chances are you will have moments when you
feel overwhelmed by those feelings which have pushed Hope to one side.
The good news is this whole day is about you and so guess what? We've got
time to feel those feelings. If you need to cry, cry. If you want to take yourself
off to bed, to hide under the duvet, then do that — but set the alarm to limit
your escape to no more than two hours.

If the weather permits, make sure you take a walk outside before it
gets dark. Walking always shifts our energy, whether we want it shifted
or not. You won't feel the same after your walk as you did when you
started out. You will feel better!

As you approach the end of the day, think back to the things that made you
feel better. Just as importantly: recognise that, even when it felt as if you
would be overwhelmed by difficult feelings, you managed to navigate them.

And so, when you finally get into bed at the end of this day
congratulate yourself.

Look, you survived!

One Week at a Time

There will be moments during this week when you suddenly realise you haven't thought about whatever happened to banish Hope. A few seconds become a few minutes become a few hours.

The 'event' and the painful feelings you've been coping with may still be very much at the forefront of your mind. But your whole thinking has adjusted because you've learned that you really do control your thoughts; and that by doing so, you can make room in your mind for other feelings and ideas.

And maybe there's even been a flash or two of Hope because trust me, she's on her way back if not already back at your side.

'Our hope that if we work hard enough and believe in ourselves, we can be whatever we dream, regardless of the limitations that others may place on us.'

Michelle Obama
FORMER FIRST LADY

Keeping Hope Alive

You could always think about Hope as being similar to a favourite houseplant.

What will happen to that plant if you go away for a while, without making arrangements for someone else to look after it?

What will happen to that plant if you forget to water or feed it; or make sure it is getting enough sunlight to make the nutrients and energy it needs
to thrive, to grow and to flower?

A neglected plant is a dead plant waiting to happen — and the same can be said for Hope.

Neglected Hopes become dead Hopes — nurtured Hopes can and will come back to life.

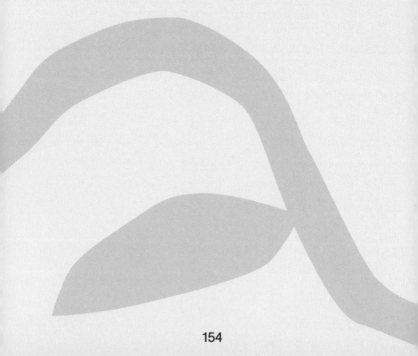

Hope fought hard to stay alive.
Even when you thought it was beaten
to nothing, burned to ashes, drowned
deep, still it flickered away, waiting
to be found again.

Juliet Marillier
AUTHOR

Change the Story

You can choose a new story for your life.

A more Hopeful one.

And ironically, the time to do that is the time when living in Hope may feel almost impossible.

If you have passed through unimaginable dark times or losses in your life, think back to those now.

What was the one thing that threw just enough light over the scene, to help you see you would not feel that way forever?

You may not have realised it until now, but the 'thing' that lit the path you took out of and away from those struggles was Hope.

Perhaps you can see then, that the greatest of all Hopes often emerge from the bleakest of struggles.

I believe there is hope for us all, even amid the suffering and maybe even inside the suffering. And that's why I write fiction, probably. It's my attempt to keep that fragile strand of radical hope, to build a fire in the darkness.

John Green
WRITER

Building Your Fire

I love this idea of building a fire to banish feelings
of hopelessness and then using Hope (capital 'H')
to fan the flames of that fire.

In the following exercise we will fan the flames of Hope with ... well,
more Hope! We're going to throw a little 'Magickal' twist into this
exercise, by writing our Hopes on a sacred herb to offer up
to the flames.

If you have a safe outdoor space where you can light a big fire
in a brazier or contained fire pit, then light one for this exercise.
If you can't have an outdoor fire and don't have an indoor stove
to burn your leaves, don't worry. You can also, with great care,
do this same exercise over a candle flame or charcoal disc.
Just make sure you take proper safety precautions; keep a dish
of water alongside the candle to drop your burning bay leaf into
if it gets too hot to hold.

Fan the flames: Before you light your fire (or candle) take time out to sit quietly. On the inside of a dried bay leaf, write down your Hopes for yourself. Use another leaf to write down your Hopes for the ones you love and another to write your Hopes for the planet.

One of the Magickal uses of bay is in manifestation. So, we are using this everyday herb to send the Hopes we desire out into the Universe where, if it is right for them to do so, they can manifest.

You won't be able to write 'War and Peace' on the bay leaves as they are quite small, so you'll need to be concise.

Once you have about half a dozen Hopes written on your Magickal leaves, offer them to the flame. Pay attention to the crackle of the dried leaves as they burn to ashes.

Remind yourself that building a fire in the darkness — either for real or as a metaphor — will give you the light you need to find your lost Hopes. In one sense, you are, literally, fanning the flames of your Hopes!

Hope is what keeps us hanging
on when we feel our rope wearing out.
A positive attitude is often the natural
result of maintaining that hope.

Lindsey Rietzsch
SINGER AND SONGWRITER

Often what feels like the end
of the world is really a challenging
pathway to a far better place.

Karen Salmansohn

SELF-HELP AUTHOR

Hope and Health

Having Hope doesn't just feel really good, it is also really, really good for your health and wellbeing.

According to academic research published in the *International Journal of Existential Psychology and Psychotherapy* in 2010, people who live in Hope report that life feels full of meaning.

The researchers, who were based at Boston University, surveyed over 500 college students to measure levels of Hope, depression and anxiety.

They returned to those same students periodically over the next few months and found that those reporting higher levels of Hope at the outset of the study had lower levels of depression and anxiety both one and two months later.

The reverse, however, was not true.

Feeling anxious or depressed does not mean Hope has gone for good and other studies have shown Hope can return, especially if we make a conscious choice to go looking for it.

Hope has also been shown to have an impact on longevity and survival, especially as we age.

In one four-year study of over 800 Americans aged between 64 and 79, the researchers found that those who had expressed higher levels of Hope at the start of the study were more likely to still be alive four years later.

In fact, 29 per cent of participants classified as 'feeling hopeless' had died, compared with just 11 per cent of those deemed more Hopeful at the start of the study.

And one of the key reasons cited for this difference in survival rates, between the Hopeful and those feeling hopeless, is that the former have been shown to make better health and lifestyle choices.

Hope and Heartache

One of the biggest challenges to Hope, whatever your life stage or personal circumstances, is heartbreak.

Few of us will live a full life and escape the pain and sorrow that comes with having your heart broken. When it feels like we will never find love again, we may even start to believe all Hope is gone.

That is never, ever true!

None of us know what lies ahead in the next day, month, or year; in our lives or the lives of those we love — and that's what makes up the magic of life.

If you want to adopt a mantra that will take you through and out the other side of heartache, borrow this one from Italian screen icon, Sophia Loren, who was no stranger to heartbreak.

According to her memoirs, she only saw her biological father a handful of times in her life, she went through a divorce and experienced two miscarriages before having her first child.

Yet the octogenarian has this to say:

'When I'm walking along in the street, I always feel that around the corner, there is something wonderful waiting for me. That's my attitude!'

Sophia Loren
ACTOR AND ACTIVIST

EXERCISE

In your Hope Journal, make a list of at least three incredible things that have already happened in your life. If you have more than three things (and how wonderful that you do) then write them all down.

And then, ask yourselves these questions:

How many of those things did you expect to happen?

How many of those things did you secretly Hope for?

How many of those things only happened because you kept on Living in Hope?

You never know what's
around the corner.

It could be everything.
Or it could be nothing.

You keep putting one foot in front of
the other and then one day, you look back
and you've climbed a mountain.

Tom Hiddleston
ACTOR

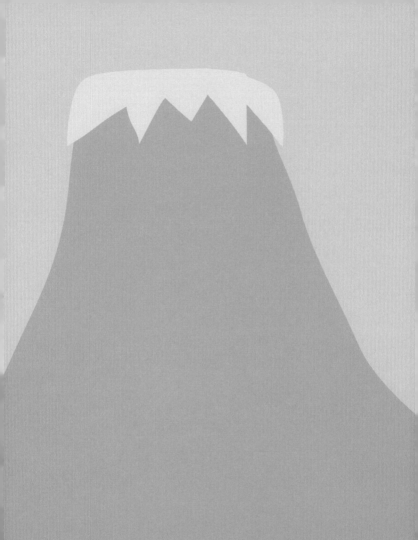

Hope and Grief

Like heartache, grief and loss are a huge challenge to your Hopes and dreams. In truth, Hope can deepen when you survive the loss of something or someone that was important to you. This could be a relationship, a job or even your youth.

Loss is a natural and inevitable part of life's rich tapestry, so there is no point fighting it.

Facing up to losses, instead of ignoring them, can actually make your life richer in the long term. And almost everyone who has reached the milestone of their fiftieth birthday will tell you the same thing.

This knowledge comes from a place of wisdom. And it is usually hard-won.

Once you begin to view grief as one of life's best teachers, you will understand how and why Hope can emerge from the greatest suffering.

It can emerge, but only if you allow it.

If you ignore the suffering, in order to guard your heart and feelings, you will damage your inner source of Hope — so, don't be tempted to do that.

When the pain feels too much and you are scared all Hope has gone, think about these words:

'I love being the age I am, because if there is enough pain or grief, I have enough experience now to realise that there's joy coming around the corner.'

They are from the American actress, Sara Gilbert, who played Darlene in the sitcom *Roseanne* in the 1980s, and who is now in her late forties.

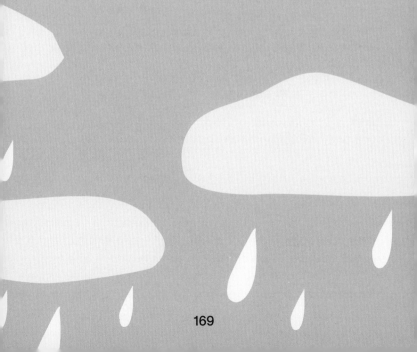

Hope is a Gift

Hope is a gift — one that is yours to share with anyone who may need it.

But how do you know what to say, to give another person more Hope?

When people are struggling to find and hang on to Hope, they don't want platitudes and they don't want to hear: 'At least ...'

'At least you have your health ...'

'At least you can try and get pregnant again...'

'At least he or she had a good long life ...'

The only person 'At least' makes feel better, is the person saying it.

To give someone Hope you need to stop pretending you can fix anything for them and just let them know that if they can hang on to Hope, things will get better.

Because they always do.

You can say something like:

I am sorry you're in pain right now, but I know things will get better for you because, in my experience, they always do.

What can I do to help you until then?

There may be nothing you can say or do, but acknowledging that someone is struggling and letting them know they're not alone can make all the difference between someone feeling Hope or despair.

All you have ...

Hope ...

Sometimes, that's
all you have

when you have
nothing else.

If you have it,
you have everything.

Unknown

Something terrible can happen
to you and yet, the day after this something
terrible, the sun still rises, and life goes on.
And therefore, so must you.

Martin Short
COMEDIAN

I believe that imagination
is stronger than knowledge.

That myth is more
potent than history.

That dreams are more powerful
than facts.

That hope always triumphs
over experience.

That laughter is the only
cure for grief.

And I believe that love is
stronger than death.

Robert Fulghum

Living Hope

'Living Hope' is a source of positive energy that is very much alive and well inside of us. It is completely crucial to our survival. If we learn to nurture this Living Hope, it will grow into a strong foundation on which we can build our lives.

The best way to Live in Hope is to connect as powerfully as we can, in the ways explored throughout this book, to the idea of Hope as something important.

We can then truly Live In Hope, supported by the inner foundation of Living Hope that we can draw on at any time.

Take a moment now to imagine all this support. Think about someone who has actively helped and supported you through a difficult experience in your life. And now imagine how Living Hope — the Hope you have inside you — is just like that helpful friend or family member.

Nobody said this is easy, but it is possible.

And when you imagine two paths opening up ahead of you — one marked Hope and the other marked hopeless, you know which one to take.

Remember, Living in Hope is always a choice.

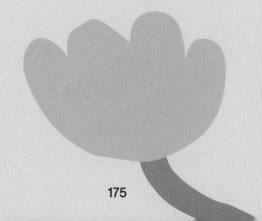

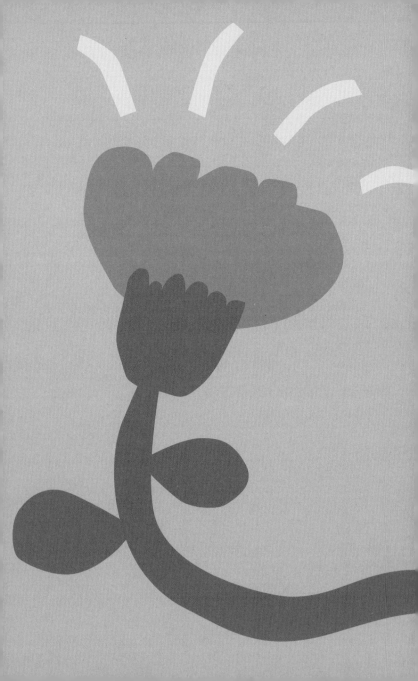

CHAPTER SIX

Hope Grows

Think of someone you know — a friend, a family member, a work colleague — who stayed Hopeful against overwhelming odds.

What do they have that keeps even the smallest flicker of Hope alive when all seems lost?

You can't see the thing they rely on to stay Hopeful, because you can't see, touch or feel Faith — with a capital 'F'.

People who have Faith know that Hope will get them through. They show the rest of us that strength comes from the courage of our convictions.

So, what if you can't see it or sell it, buy it or bottle it?

That doesn't mean it — Faith — doesn't exist.

Never lose hope

Storms make people stronger,
and never last forever.

Roy T. Bennett
AUTHOR

Plant seeds of Happiness,
Hope, Success, and Love;
It will all come back
to you in abundance.
This is the law of nature.

Steve Maraboli
MOTIVATIONAL SPEAKER

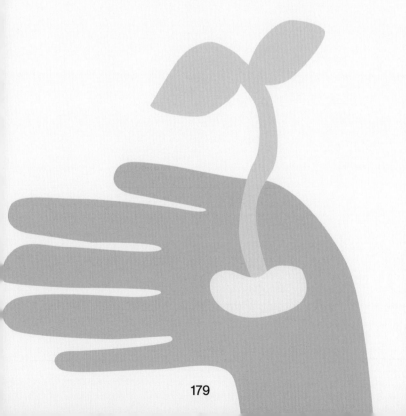

The Law of Nature

Let's get this idea really ingrained as a lifelong philosophy: plant the right seeds and you'll get the right rewards.

And if this is a law of nature, then planting Hope to get more Hope in the future is an inevitability.

Like the sun rising each morning, regardless of what's happened the day before.

Like a tiny acorn becoming an ancient oak tree — given time and the right conditions to thrive.

There are other 'natural' laws that tell us that if we choose Hope and we plant Hope then Hope will grow.
These include:

The Law of Attraction

The Law of Polarity

The Law of Relativity

The Law of Cause and Effect

The Law of Rhythm

The Law of Perpetual
Transmutation
of Energy

The Law Of Attraction =
Like Attracts Like

Simple but elegant, this natural law tells us we will attract people who share the same energy we project. So, when it comes to Hope, this means Hopeful People attract ...
MORE HOPEFUL PEOPLE.

All your thoughts are energy. All your feelings are energy. Everything you say, do and think is energy.

And so, just like a magnet, that energy of yours attracts or repels other types of energy.

Another way to think about this energy is to think about it as your 'vibe'.

The Law of Attraction states that you will attract what you give out — so if you want more Hope and more Hopeful People in your life, what do you have to decide to do?

You have to decide to practice being a more Hopeful person yourself.

We've already seen Hope is a choice and we've learned, in earlier chapters, how we can so easily make that our choice.

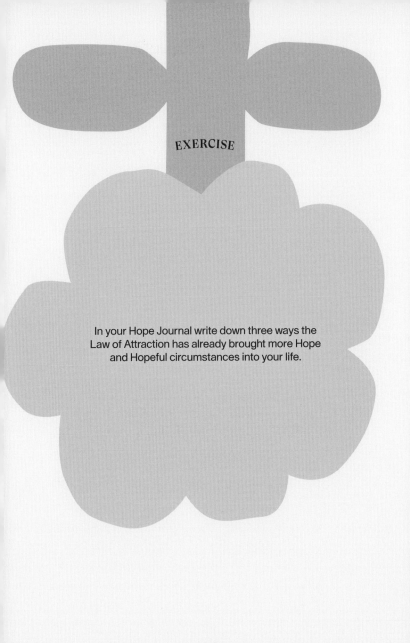

EXERCISE

In your Hope Journal write down three ways the Law of Attraction has already brought more Hope and Hopeful circumstances into your life.

The Law Of Polarity =
Everything In The Universe Has
An Equal And Exact Opposite

What's the equal and exact opposite of Hope?

Feeling hopeless.

We've seen throughout this book just how powerful Hope can be; which means that if you apply the Law of Polarity, hopelessness must be just as powerful.

Therapists will tell you the most difficult state of mind to treat successfully, and for a person to overcome, are intense feelings of hopelessness.

When you are full of Hope, you want to leap out of bed in the morning, eager to start your day.

When you are full of hopelessness, you want to stay under the duvet and your only Hope is that the world will go away.

In your Hope Journal, write down three ways the Law of Polarity has already impacted your life. Have there been times when your Hopes were dashed, only to be replaced by equally powerful feelings of hopelessness?

The Law Of Relativity =
Everything is Relative!

This law tells us you cannot define or really understand something without a comparison.

Your mind automatically makes comparisons with people around you. This is a perfectly natural biosocial mechanism; your brain wants to understand where you fit in relation to the external world and other people. But constant measuring can feel competitive and toxic because your mind will usually imagine others as being much, much, better off than you.

The trick to overcoming this tendency is to train your mind not to make comparisons to other people; but to make comparisons between the 'now' you and 'past' you.

Go back as far as you like in your personal history with this comparison.

It will take practice, but every time your mind starts to compare you to another person; remind it to measure you against yourself and your own unique Hopes and dreams.

In your Hope Journal, write down the names of three people you know and next to them, write three things you imagine they have so much more of than you.

Love? Money? Happiness? Friends? Hope?

Now, put a line through those imaginings.
A thick strikeout line!

Write down three things you already have and alongside that list, write three additional things you Hope for.

Love? Money? Happiness? Friends? Hope?

Can you see how this simple exercise eliminates the competitive element of the law of relativity and adjusts your mindset? You are now thinking about what you have, and not about how much better off someone else is compared to you.

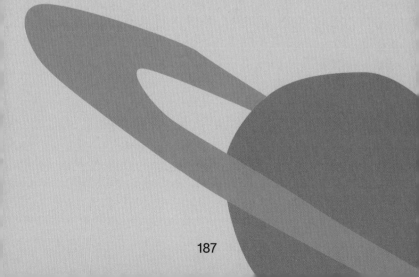

The Law Of Cause and Effect = For Every Action There Is An Effect

Chances are you already know and already think about this natural law but it's worth reminding ourselves that, for every action there is a subsequent reaction that ripples out into the Universe.

Your actions will impact everyone around you and everyone around them.

That means if you behave in a Hopeful way you will be encouraging others to do the same and before you know it, Hope has grown not only in your own immediate circles but wider ones too.

The Law Of Rhythm =
Everything in the universe is
moving in perfect rhythm

Think about the movements of a pendulum swinging rhythmically back and forth.

The Law of Rhythm tells us that for every up movement there will be one down; for every advance, a retreat; and for every swing to the left, a swing back to the right. The Universe works hard to keep an even keel.

Knowing this allows us to hang on to Hope because we understand that life itself ebbs and flows and that our own lives are no different.

We may lose Hope for a while but one day, we will regain Hope.

That's the Law of Nature!

The Law Of Perpetual Transmutation of Energy = Nothing stays the same

It is a natural law that you cannot destroy or create new energy — what you can do is transmute it into something else. This means that nothing lasts forever or stays the same forever. So, if your Hope has taken a battering and you find yourself losing it, remind yourself it won't be this way forever!

You may not realise you are already a wizard at transmuting energy, but you are! There is a simple thing you can do to prove it to yourself — walking.

This simple everyday activity unlocks your energy when you choose to do it mindfully and, by doing so, changes (transmutes) your state of mind. You may have felt negative when you stepped outside the front door but you will feel more positive when you return because you have changed the energy.

EXERCISE

Go for an hour-long walk. Take your phone in case you need it but keep it in your pocket. Walk alone (or with a dog) and don't walk with headphones.

Pay attention to everything you see. What do you feel on your skin? What can you smell? Is it quiet? Is it noisy? How does it feel to keep putting one foot in front of the other?

Spiritual healers will often use the
phrase 'change the energy, change the outcome.'
And now you know that you can also transmute
energy to grow Hope in your life — all you have
to do is keep your attention focused on it.

Keep this little book close by for inspiration,
and to remind yourself of all the ways in which
you can keep Hope alive.

Hope is a match in a dark tunnel,
a moment of light, just enough to reveal the
path ahead and ultimately the way out.

Unknown

There is no despair so absolute as that which comes with the first moments of our first great sorrow, when we have not yet known what it is to have suffered and be healed, to have despaired and have recovered hope.

George Eliot
NOVELIST

Hope Overcomes Despair

A remarkable study carried out in 2015 showed how Hope can lift people permanently out of poverty.

Researchers followed the lives of over 20,000 impoverished people living in Ethiopia, Ghana, Honduras, India, Pakistan and Peru, and found that giving people a resource gave them Hope for a better future.

The resource, in this instance, was a cow.

After receiving the cow, the families were shown how to look after it.

Before long, something unexpected came into the mix: Hope.

Armed with the cow, as well as the skills to care for the animal; the people taking part in the study reported that they finally had the Hope of a much better future.

The researchers concluded it was Hope, and not charity or money, that helped them improve their lives in the long term.

This study teaches us all something important — that often our Hope is linked with our resources (by which I don't mean money).

EXERCISE

In your Hope Journal, make a list of your resources (excluding money).

These may include:

Your coping skills

Your ability to self-reflect

Your self-belief

Your ability to go looking for Hope when it disappears during a crisis

Knowing how to empower yourself

Surrounding yourself with Hopeful role models

Remembering your successes and achievements to date

Now, read over this long list. How much better do you feel about yourself?

How much more Hopeful do you feel about your future, now you've remembered the resources at your disposal?

Shared Hope Always Grows

From campaigns like Black Lives Matter to MeToo and Take Back The Night, even the hardest-hitting of social and political campaigns have Hope at their heart — the shared Hope that together we can make things better and safer for everyone.

What happens if I bring my Hope to the meeting about changing attitudes to how we use our finite planetary resources? And I add it to your Hope that we can and will make a difference?

What happens when we then unleash this double dose of Hope — yours and mine — into a campaign where tens, and then hundreds and then thousands, agree to share their Hope and vision for a better way of doing things?

What happens is that Hope grows exponentially — which really just means Hope grows really fast.

EXERCISE

Choose one of your Hopes that you believe can make a difference to the lives of many. This could be about protecting the planet or animals or children or any other vulnerable group.

Now find a local group that campaigns in some way to help bring about the improvements you are imagining.

Find a group whose values (and ways of campaigning) align with yours and see how quickly you recognise Hope in all the actions the group agrees to take.

If you can't find a local group that shares your values, then start one. Take that first Hopeful step and see where it leads and how your shared mission grows.

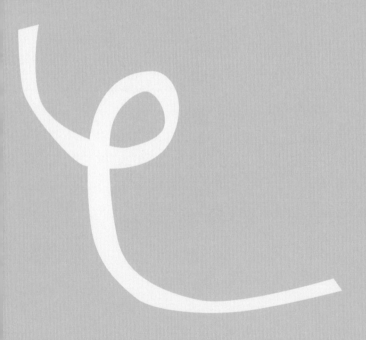

Never doubt that a small
group of thoughtful, committed citizens
can change the world; indeed, it is the
only thing that ever has.

Margaret Mead
ENVIRONMENTALIST

Embodied Hope

Nelson Mandela (1918—2013) was the South African anti-apartheid political leader, revolutionary and inspiring philanthropist who served as that countries' first black president from 1994—1999.

He had been incarcerated in 1962 and was kept in prison for 27 years, accused of trying to overthrow the state.

Mandela came to embody the universal aspirations of dispossessed people from around the world — their Hopes, not only for a better life, but also a moral transformation in the way we conduct our affairs.

'I never lost hope that this great transformation would occur,' he said.

'I always knew that deep down in every human heart, there is mercy and generosity.'

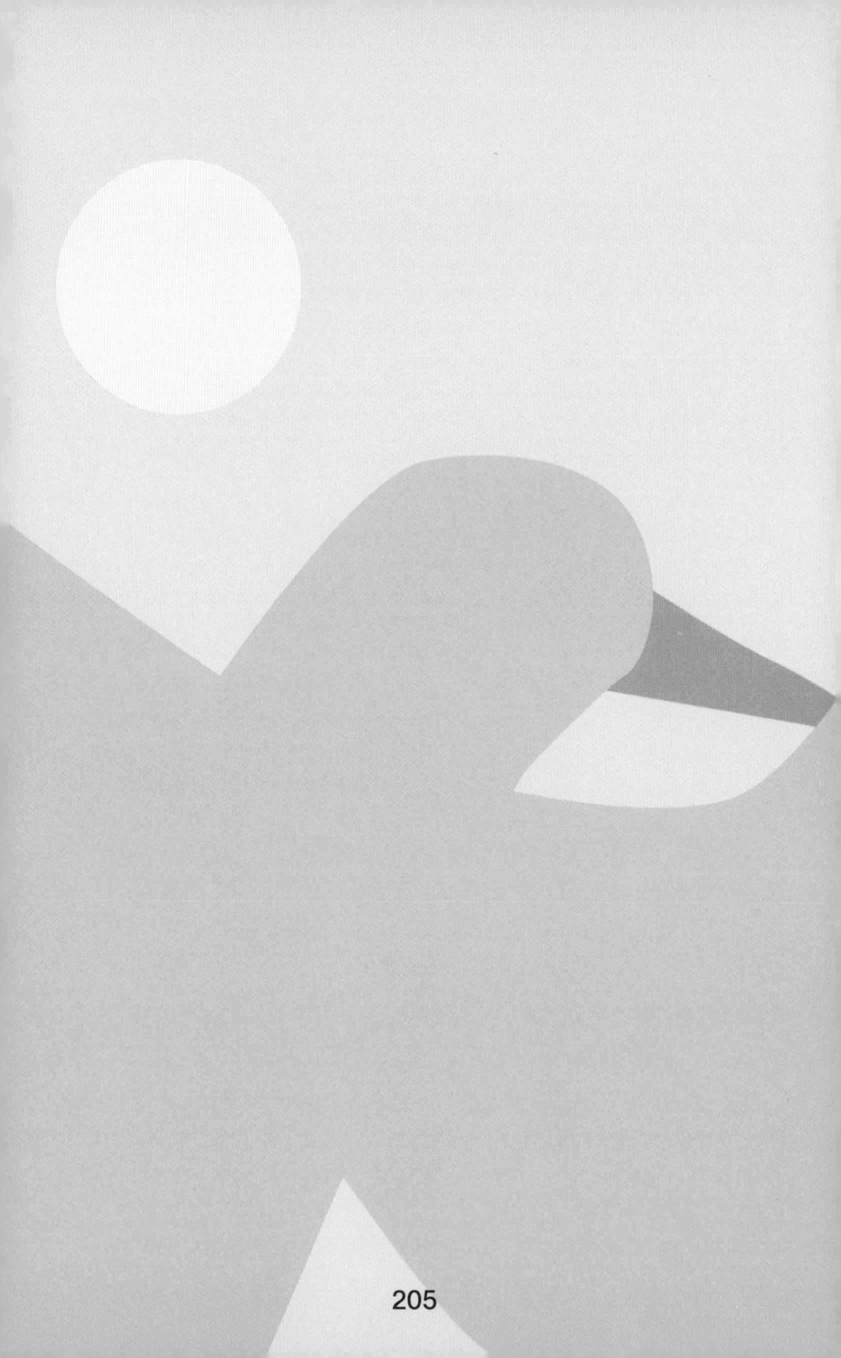

A Daily Hope Prayer

In this beautiful, three-step Morning Prayer from the Native American tradition, we learn to 'plant' ourselves in Hope and Gratitude for each and every new day.

This tradition uses the term 'Creator God' to refer to divinity, but you don't need to be religious or believe in a specific god to use this prayer.

You can easily change the words to suit your own spiritual preferences; for example, use the terms Mother Earth or Nature or The Universe.

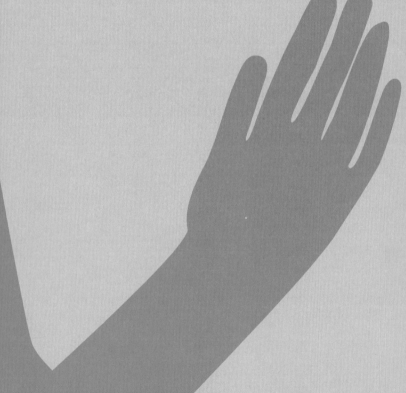

First step:

Plant your feet firmly on the Earth. Using your five senses, give thanks to our Creator God for the countless ways God comes to us through creation — for all the beauty that your eyes see, for all the sounds that your ears ear, for all the scents that you smell, the tastes that you taste, for all that you feel (the sun, wind, rain, snow; warm or cold). Pray this day that you may be open and attuned to the countless ways that our Creator God comes to us through your senses, through the gifts of creation.

Second Step:

Let go of all the pain, struggle, regret, failures, garbage of yesterday — step out of it — leave it behind; brush the dust of it from your feet.

Third Step:

With this third and final step, step into the gift of the new day, full of Hope, promise, and potential. Give thanks for the gift of this new day, which God has made!
Amen.

Jose Hobday
SIMPLE LIVING TEACHER

There was never a night or a problem that could defeat sunrise or hope.

Bernard Williams
PHILOSOPHER

It is in collectivities that
we find reservoirs of hope
and optimism.

Angela Davis

PHILOSOPHER

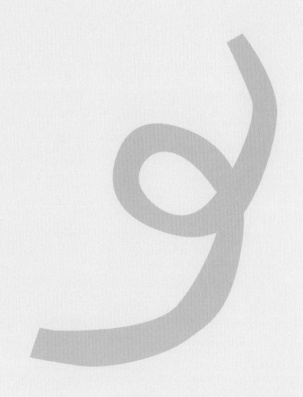

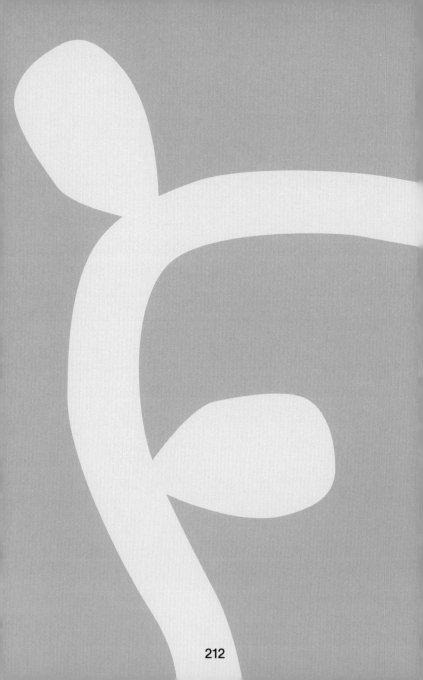

AFFIRMATION

In your Hope Journal make
this affirmation in writing.

I am on the path I am meant to be on.

There are always better things ahead.

I am stronger than any challenge
that comes my way.

I have enough Hope to carry me
through the tough times.

I have enough Hope to
share with others.

H.O.P.E.

H is for Hanging on to Hope.

O is for Overcoming All Obstacles.

P is for Protecting Hope.

E is for Transmuting
Your Energy Into Hope.

Life is Beautiful ...
Its beauty lies in Hope
Hope of success
Hope of happiness
Hope of prosperity
Hope of Life.

Alisha
INFLUENCER

Never let go of Hope.
One day you will see that
it has all finally come together.
What you have always wished
for has finally come to be.
You will look back and laugh
at what has passed and you
will ask yourself ... 'How did
I get through all of that?'

Unknown

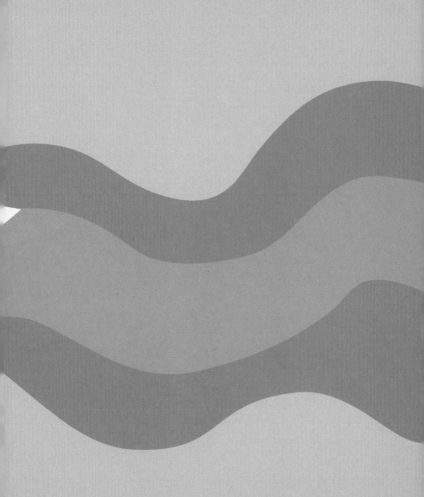

How did you get through?

You already know that answer ...

Harvest Time

In all life cycles there is a time to sow, a time to grow and a time to harvest.

Martin Luther King once said that nothing was ever done in this world that was not done with Hope. He is right, some of the most important things that have happened in the world have been accomplished by people who just refused to give up; who kept trying even when it seemed all Hope was gone.

Hope is never gone.

It may be dormant. It may be just a quiet whisper, waiting patiently to be invited into your life.

But open the door, let Hope in and you will find the courage to live the authentic life you Hope for and to live your life to the full.

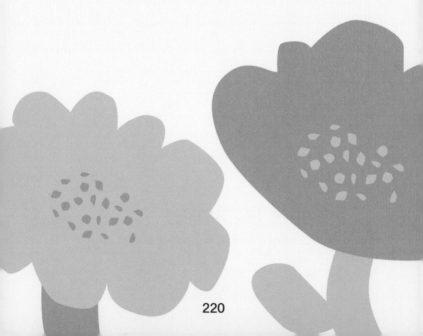

If you only carry one thing throughout
your entire life let it be Hope.

Let it be Hope that better
things are always ahead.

Let it be Hope that you can get through
even the toughest of times.

Let it be Hope that you are stronger than
any challenge that comes your way.

Let it be Hope that you are exactly
where you are meant to be right now,
and that you are on the path to where
you are meant to be ...

Because during these times,
Hope will be the very thing
that carries you through.

Nikki Banas
POET

Acknowledgements

With thanks to my publisher, Kate Pollard, for steering her vision of a book that will inspire Hope in all who read it my way. And to our editor, Jo Hanks, for her attention to diversity and detail, and the design team at Evi O. Studio.

And on a personal note, my forever thanks to Chris and Rachel – true champions of Hope in my life through one of the most challenging times and in the lives of many others!

About the Author

Susan Elizabeth Clark is a self-help writer who specialises in shining a light on those topics that can help people overcome their challenges to live their best lives. She has studied esoteric traditions and yoga in both India and the UK. Susan lives in Yorkshire.

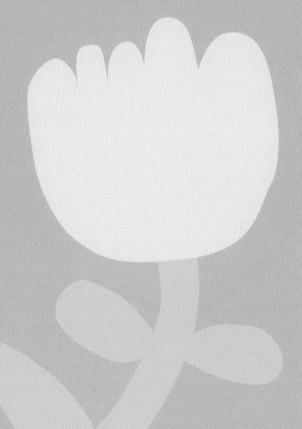

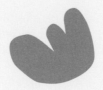

Published by OH Editions
20 Mortimer Street
London W1T 3JW

Design © 2021 OH Editions

ISBN 978-1-914317-00-2

Text © Susan Elizabeth Clark
Editorial: Jo Hanks
Design and illustrations: Evi-O.Studio | Kait Polkinghorne & Susan Le
Production: Rachel Burgess

A CIP catalogue record for this book is available
from the British Library

Printed and bound in China

10 9 8 7 6 5 4 3 2 1